Annil Dhingra
Saurabh Harkanwal Kaur Bhullar

Root Apex & Its Significance In Endodontics

AF154037

Annil Dhingra
Saurabh Harkanwal Kaur Bhullar

Root Apex & Its Significance In Endodontics

LAP LAMBERT Academic Publishing

Impressum / Imprint

Bibliografische Information der Deutschen Nationalbibliothek: Die Deutsche Nationalbibliothek verzeichnet diese Publikation in der Deutschen Nationalbibliografie; detaillierte bibliografische Daten sind im Internet über http://dnb.d-nb.de abrufbar.
Alle in diesem Buch genannten Marken und Produktnamen unterliegen warenzeichen-, marken- oder patentrechtlichem Schutz bzw. sind Warenzeichen oder eingetragene Warenzeichen der jeweiligen Inhaber. Die Wiedergabe von Marken, Produktnamen, Gebrauchsnamen, Handelsnamen, Warenbezeichnungen u.s.w. in diesem Werk berechtigt auch ohne besondere Kennzeichnung nicht zu der Annahme, dass solche Namen im Sinne der Warenzeichen- und Markenschutzgesetzgebung als frei zu betrachten wären und daher von jedermann benutzt werden dürften.

Bibliographic information published by the Deutsche Nationalbibliothek: The Deutsche Nationalbibliothek lists this publication in the Deutsche Nationalbibliografie; detailed bibliographic data are available in the Internet at http://dnb.d-nb.de.
Any brand names and product names mentioned in this book are subject to trademark, brand or patent protection and are trademarks or registered trademarks of their respective holders. The use of brand names, product names, common names, trade names, product descriptions etc. even without a particular marking in this work is in no way to be construed to mean that such names may be regarded as unrestricted in respect of trademark and brand protection legislation and could thus be used by anyone.

Coverbild / Cover image: www.ingimage.com

Verlag / Publisher:
LAP LAMBERT Academic Publishing
ist ein Imprint der / is a trademark of
OmniScriptum GmbH & Co. KG
Heinrich-Böcking-Str. 6-8, 66121 Saarbrücken, Deutschland / Germany
Email: info@lap-publishing.com

Herstellung: siehe letzte Seite /
Printed at: see last page
ISBN: 978-3-659-63830-5

ROOT APEX & ITS SIGNIFICANCE IN ENDODONTICS

DR ANNIL DHINGRA

PROFESSOR & HEAD

DR. HAKANWAL KAUR BHULLAR

P.G. STUDENT

DR. SAURABH

P.G. STUDENT

DEPARTMENT OF CONSERVATIVE
DENTISTRY AND ENDODONTICS

D.J. COLLEGE OF DENTAL SCIENCE AND
RESEARCH

MODINAGAR, U.P. INDIA

ROOT APEX & ITS SIGNIFICANCE IN ENDODONTICS

TABLE OF CONTENT

Chapter 1

INTRODUCTION

Root canal system is one of the most complex topics in the study of human anatomy. Its internal complexity is often concealed by the relative simplicity and uniformity of external surface of the root. The terminal part of root canal is the most complex and most significant part. The root apex and the tissue that surround it are the center of most activity and concern in the treatment and filling of root canal.

Because the stages of root development and the type of tissue present within the roots of teeth are significant, the root apex is of considerable interest to the endodontists. For successful treatment of root canal, a practitioner should have good knowledge of the architecture of the root apex and its variance, ability to analyze the radiographs

correctly, and to feel it through tactile sensation during instrumentation.

From the early work of Hess and Zurcher published in the 1920s to the most recent studies showing anatomic complexities of the root canal system, it has long been established that a root with a tapering canal and a single foremen is the exception rather than the rule. Multiple foramina, additional canals, fins, deltas, intercanal connections, loops, C-shaped canals, and accessory canals have been reported by many authors. Consequently, the practitioner must treat each tooth assuming that complex anatomy occurs often enough to be considered normal.

One of the most controversial issues in root canal therapy is the apical limit of root canal instrumentation and obturation. For decades, this subject has been discussed among endodontists. The related literature often creates confusion and uncertainty for those looking for adequate clinical solutions based on facts rather than on notions. Little importance has been given to the detailed anatomy of this region and, particularly to the position and topography of the apical canal constriction.

Chapter 2

Development of Root Apex

The root begins to develop after the enamel and the dentin formation has reached the future cementoenamel junction. The outer and inner enamel epithelia begin to proliferate and come together to form a sort of diaphragm facing the interior of the structure, which will become the pulp cavity or the root canal. When this cellular diaphragm is formed, the stage of formation of Hertwig's epithelial root sheath (HERS)is reached.

HERS consists of only the outer and inner enamel epithelia ;therefore it does not include the stratum intermedium and stellate reticulum. HERS shapes the roots and initiates radicular dentine formation.

Root sheath proliferates horizontally towards the dental papilla to form the epithelial diaphragm. This process partially encloses the dental papilla and delineates the apical foramen. Soon the ectomesenchymal cells of dental papilla, which are present above the epithelial diaphragm, start proliferating and deposition of root dentin occurs. The plane of the diaphragm remains relatively fixed during the development and growth of the root. The free end of the diaphragm does not develop into the connective tissue, but the epithelium proliferates coronally to the epithelial diaphragm.

Odontoblasts differentiation and dentin formation follow the lengthening of the root sheath. According to Orban, the epithelial diaphragm (i.e. future root apex) remains in place whereas the tooth crown and supporting structures move occlusally. After the dentin is deposited to the entire length of the root, the HERS split to allow the cells of the dental sac to come in contact with the dentin. These cells get differentiated into cement blasts and start depositing cementum on radicular dentin.

Two types of cementum are deposited on the root. If the cementoblasts retract while cementum is laid down, the tissue formed is known as a cellular cementum. If cementoblasts do not retract and get entrapped by new cementum, the tissue formed is known as cellular cementum and the trapped cementoblasts are called cementocytes.

Acellular cementum is formed around the coronal and middle third of root whereas cellular cementum is formed at the apical third of the root with alternating layers of acellular cementum. This slow deposition of the cementum continues throughout the life and makes the layer of cementum at the apical third of the root thicker than cervical third, which maintains the length of the tooth, constricts the apical foramen, and deviates the apical foramen from the centre of the apex.

The remnant epithelial cell clusters formed as a result of breakup of HERS migrate towards the dental sac. They remain in the periodontal ligament close to the surface of cementum. These cells are called cell rests of Malassez. When they are stimulated, they have the potential to differentiate into any cell as the need arises. The rapid sequence of proliferation and destruction of HERS explain the fact that it cannot be seen as a continuous layer on the surface of the developing root.

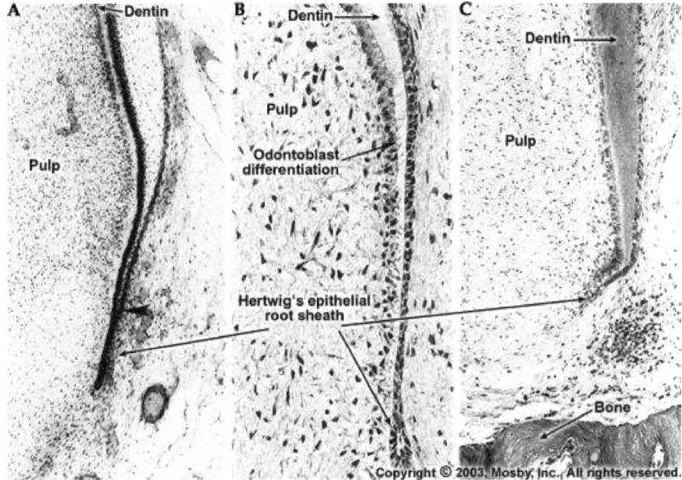

Figure 1: Root formation. (A) The root begins to form as an extension of the inner and outer dental epithelia in the cervical loop region (arrowhead), which forms a bilayered structure called HERS. The root sheath induces differentiation of odontoblasts from the radicular pulp. (B) The differentiation of odontoblasts and the formation of root dentin. (C) Root formation is almost complete. The root sheath is now a small tag of epithelium inducing the final differentiation of odontoblasts at the rim of the future apical foramen.

The cementum, periodontal ligament, and the alveolar bone are derived from the dental sac. In fact, the mesenchyme of the dental sac produces a large number of collagen fibres (to form the future periodontal ligament), as well as the organic matrix of the bone (alveolar bone) and the cementum.

This matrix is deposited around the previously formed collagen fibre bundles and subsequently mineralizes. This explains the presence of fibres embedded in the hard tissues at each end, bone, and cementum, where they are known as Sharpey's fibres. The alveolar bone and the cementum develop around these fibres, thus anchoring the dental structure to the surrounding alveolar bone.

SINGLE AND MULTIPLEROOT FORMATION

The horizontal diaphragm or HERS may vary in shape, depending on whether the teeth are single or multiple rooted. In fact, the diaphragm's shape determines the number of roots in a tooth.

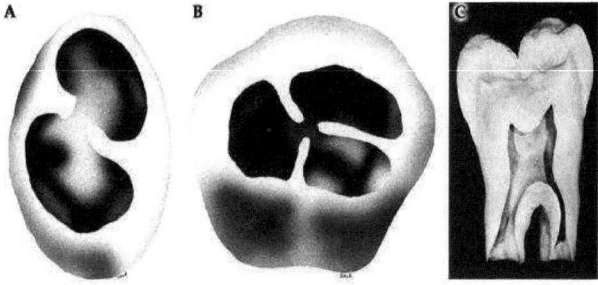

Figure 2:

The wide apical foramen is reduced first to the width of the diaphragmatic opening itself and later it is further narrowed by opposition of dentin and cementum to the apex of the root. Differential growth of the epithelial diaphragm in multi-rooted teeth leads to the division of the root track into two or three roots.

During the general growth of the enamel, the cervical opening expands in such a way that long tongue-like extensions of the horizontal diaphragm appear. Two such extensions are found in the germs of lower molars and three in the germs of upper molars.

Before division of the root trunk takes place, the free ends of these horizontal epithelial flags grow towards each other and fuse. The single cervical opening of the coronal enamel organ is then divided into two or three openings.

Dentin formation begins on the pulpal surface of the dividing epithelial bridges. Root development follows in the same way as described for single rooted teeth on the periphery of each opening.

FORMATION OF LATERAL CANALS

Sometimes, small portions of Hertwig's vertical root sheath disappear before the odontoblast differentiation. This small island of "lack of cells" of HERS, where odontoblasts do not differentiate and thus dentin does not form, is responsible for the formation of lateral canal.

According to Weinmann, "the development of all the lateral branches of the root canals may be a defect of the epithelial root sheath of Hertwig which occurs during the development of the root because of the presence of a large, supernumerary blood vessel". As a result, if the root sheath formation is interrupted before the formation of the dentin, a defect in the dentinal wall occurs. This defect can be observed at the floor of the pulp chamber of a multi-rooted tooth if the union of the tongue-like extensions of the epithelial diaphragm is incomplete because of the presence of a vessel.

The lateral canals formation is attributed to the entrapment of vessels of the periodontal plexus that course around and within the apex of the developing tooth within Hertwig's membrane.

To elucidate the high incidence of accessory canals near the root tip, Cutright and Baskar cite Kovacs that once the tooth enters occlusion, the tip of the root grows within the alveolar bone rather than growing outwardly.

According to this theory, each time the vessels of the periodontal plexus are forced to curve apically and then coronally to enter the apex, there is a high probability that they will remain entrapped in HERS and then be surrounded by dentin. In the furcation area of multi-rooted teeth, the origin of the accessory canals is also attributed to vessels of the periodontal plexus that remain entrapped at the points of fusion of the tongue-like extensions.

ROOT LENGTH AND APICAL CLOSURE

One should have the knowledge about the dates of tooth eruption and the completion of the root length and apical closure because root formation and apical closure havean important function in the repair of inflamed dental pulps after endodontic therapy.

Tooth	Emergence into oral cavity	Completion of root length (years)		Apical closure (years)	
		Male	Female	Male	Female
Upper 1st incisor	7–8	10 ¾	10	–	–
Upper 2nd incisor	8–9	12	11 ¼	–	–
Lower 1st incisor	6–7	8 ¾	8 ½	10	9 ½
Lower 2nd incisor	7–8	10	9 ½	11 ½	10 ½
Lower canine	9–10	12 ½	11	18	14
Lower 1st premolar	10–12	13	12	16 ½	15
Lower 2nd premolar	11–12	14	13	17 ½	16 ¾
Lower 1st molar	6–7	Mesial root 7	7	10 ½	9 ¾
		Distal root 7½	7 ½	10 ¾	11
Lower 2nd molar	11–13	14	13	16	13
		14 ½	13 ¾	18	17 ¾
Lower 3rd molar	17–21	20	20 ¾	23 ½	24 ½
		20 ½	21	24 ½	25 ¼

Clinical significance

A young, incompletely formed root has a funnel-shaped opening exists at apex,which contains connective tissue, blood vessels, and nerves that enters and exit the root canals. Therefore, successful repair of inflamed dental pulps is observed in teeth with incomplete apical closure when compared with the teeth with completed apical closure. This may be possibly due to the unobstructed metabolism.

Chapter 3

Anatomy and Histology of the Root Apex

The anatomic apex is the tip or the end of root is determined morphologically whereas radiographic apex is the tip or end of root is determined radiographically. The location of the radiographic apex may vary from the anatomic apex due to root morphology and radiographic distortion.

The classic concept of apical root anatomy is based on three anatomic and histologic landmarks – the apical constriction (AC), the cementodentinal junction (CDJ), and the apical foramen (AF).

The AFis "circumference or rounded edge, like a funnelor crater, that differentiates the termination of the cemental canal from the exterior surface of the root. It is an aperture at or near the apex of root, through which the nerve and blood vessels of pulp pass. Thus, the AF represents the junction of the pulp and periodontal tissue. In a young, incompletely developed tooth, the AF is shaped like a funnel, with the wider portion extending outside. That is why it is often called blunderbuss apex. The site and shape of the fully formed foramen vary in each tooth and in the same tooth at different periods of time. AF may be round, oval or elliptical, or semilunar in shape.

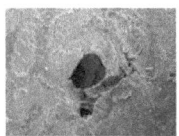 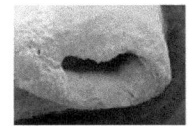 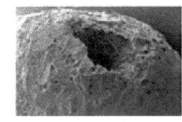

The AF is not always located at the centre of the root apex. It is a myth that the AF coincides with the anatomical apex of the tooth. This is rare, and usually the AF opens 0.5–1.0 mm from the anatomical apex. This distance is not always equal and may increase as the tooth ages because of the deposition of secondary cementum on the outer surface of the root and the deposition of secondary dentine on the walls of the root canal. The AF may exit on the mesial, distal, labial, or lingual surface of the root, and usually slightly eccentrically

This apical portion of the root canal having narrowest diameter is called *apical constriction*. It occurs approximately 0.5–1.0 mm from the AF; it is also called *minor apicaldiameter*. Postoperative discomfort is generally greater when this area is violated by instruments or filling materials and the healing process may be compromise. Again, the portion of the AC differs with age, as stated earlier. The root filling should stop at this constriction as it could serve as "apical dentine matrix."

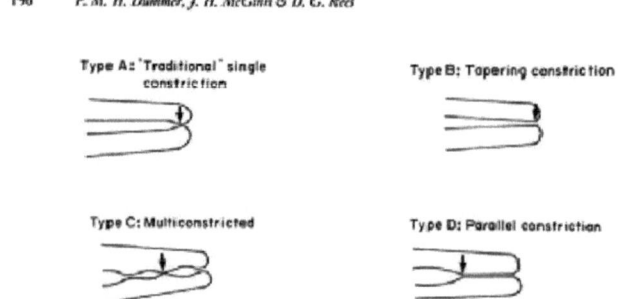

196   P. M. H. Dummer, J. H. McGinn & D. G. Rees

Fig. 3. Classification of apical constrictions. *Arrow* indicates narrowest portion of canal and point of measurement.

Figure 2: Apical constriction. Narrower portion of canal and point of measurement are indicated by arrows.

Above several shapes of apical "constriction" are given by Dummer *et al.*: parallel (35%), single (18%), tapering/"classic" (15%), flaring (18%), delta (12%).

The space present between the major and minor diameters has been described as funnel shaped or hyperbolic, or as having the shape of a morning glory. In a young person, the mean distance between the major

13

and minor apical diameters is 0.5 mm and it is 0.67 mm in an elderly person.

The *cemetodentinal junction* is the point in the canal where cementum interacts with dentine. It is also the point where pulp tissue ends and periodontal tissue begins. The location of CDJ in the root canal varies considerably. It is generally not the same area as the AC and generally approximately 1 mm from the AF. Cementum reaches the same level on all canal walls only 5% of the time. The greatest extension generally occurs on the concave side of the canal curvature. This variability reconfirmed that the CDJ and AC are generally not the same area and that the CDJ should be considered just a point at which two histologic tissues interact within the root canal. The diameter of the canal at the CDJ was highly irregular and was found to be 353□mm for maxillary centrals, 292 mm for lateral incisors, and 298 mm for canines.

Kuttler (1955) concluded that the root canal has two main sections, a longer conical section in the coronal region consisting of dentine and a shorter funnel-shaped section consisting of cementum located in the apical portion. The shape of this apical portion is considered to be an inverted cone; its base being located at the major AF. The apex of the inverted cone is the minor foramen that is often thought to coincide with the AC regarded as being at or near the CDJ. In other words, the most apical portion of the root canal system narrows from the opening of the major foramen, which is within cementum, to a constriction (minor foramen) before widening out in the main canal to produce an hourglass shape.

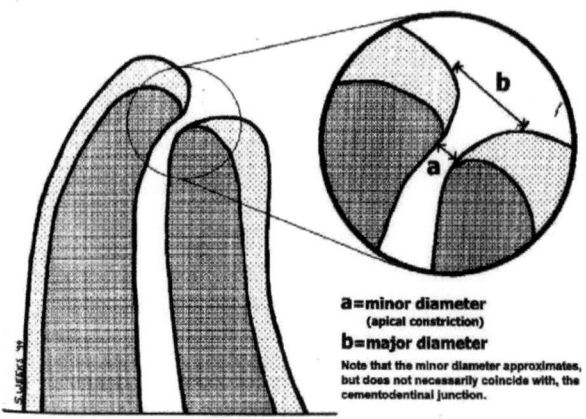

Figure 3: Schematic diagram showing anatomic features of root apex

*Accessory canals*are channels that lead from the radicular pulplaterally via the root dentine to the periodontal tissue. They may be seen anywhere along the root dentine, but particularly numerous at apical third; some of them open approximately at right angles to the main pulp cavity and are termed "lateral canals." Lateral canals are found more in the roots of posterior teeth and occasionally in the roots of anterior teeth, which is more common in bifurcation and trifurcations regions of molar teeth.

Hess in 1925, using vulcanite corrosion specimens, reported the incidence of 16.9% of lateral canals in all teeth. According to him accessory foramina have a mean diameter of 6–60 μm. In many teeth, the width of the accessory canals and sometimes lateral canals is small, allowing for only small calibre blood vessels and their supporting stroma. Generally, these small canals cannot be observed on X-rays, if the root

canal breaks up into multiple tiny canals, it is called as delta system because of its complexity.

In many teeth with a fused root, a web-like connection, which can be complete or incomplete, is observed between two canals and is called isthmus. An *isthmus* is a narrow, ribbon-shaped communication between two root canals that contain pulp or tissues derived from the pulp. It is called a corridor by green, lateral connection pineda and anastomosis by vertucci. Isthmuses often merge two canals into one at 3 mm from the apex. Thus, the isthmus is a part of the canal system and not a separate entity, so it must be cleaned, shaped, and retroseal accordingly because it can function as a reservoir of bacteria. Kim and Kratchman (2006) identified five types of isthmuses that can be found on a bevelled root surface.

Type 1: It is a barely traceable communication between two canals, classified as an incomplete isthmus.

Type 2: It is a definite connection between two main canals. Type 2 complete isthmus can be a straight line between two canals. It is a C-shaped connection.

Type 3: It is a complete but very short connection between two canals and looks like one elongated canal.

Type 4: It can be complete or incomplete, but it connects three or more canals rather than two.

Type 5: It includes two or three canal openings on an elongated, ovoid root surface; these do not have any visible connection even after being stained. Weather to treat it as isthmus to connect the canal or to treat the orifice only is the dilemma faced by professionals while treating the root surface.

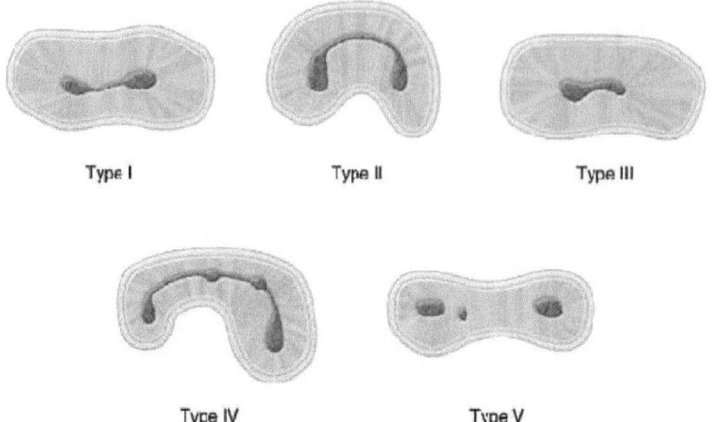

Type I   Type II   Type III

Type IV   Type V

HISTOLOGY OF APICAL THIRD

The connective tissue of the root canal, foramen, and the periradicular zone forms an inseparable tissue continuum at the periapex. This intimate relationship is confirmed by the frequency of disease in the pulp, initiating disease beyond the tooth. Immediate therapy must often focus on the periradicular region when both the pulp and periapex are jointly involved. More commonly, only pulp therapy is required. Healing of the periradicular tissue generally occurs spontaneously, showing its capacity to repair. During preparation of the pulp space, the cardinal principles of instrumentation and obturation, aimed at

Confining everything to the canal space, indicate that it is very important to respect the periradicular connective tissue.

Dentinogenesis is uninterrupted from the crown throughout the length of the root. The process is same for both the crown and the root except for the differences given below:

17

1. Radicular dentine matrix is deposited against the root sheath, instead of ameloblasts.

2. Dentinal tubule is different in the path of the root.

3. Dentine is covered by cementum in the root.

4. Dentine forms most of the root tissue, except at the apices of the older teeth in which the tips may be composed of cementum only.

APICAL DENTINE

In the apical region, the odontoblasts of the pulp are absent or flattened or cuboidal in shape. The produced dentine is not as tubular as the coronal dentine but is more amorphous and irregular. This type of dentine is known as sclerotic dentine. Its amount generally increases with age. The sclerotic bands are narrower towards the root canal and they fan out towards the mesial and distal root surfaces in a butterfly pattern.

The use of isotopes has shown that the secondary mineralization of sclerotic dentine is characterized by a prolonged period of crystal deposition at a considerable distance from the pulp cells. This intratubular process leads to a high micro radiographic density much greater than that of intertubular dentine. The extent of mineralization of the sclerotic dentinal tubules approximates that of cementum or peritubular dentine. The sclerotic zone contains tubule-free dentine near the root canal. The dentinal tubules become partially or completely obliterated.

The dentine becomes optically transparent, being uniform enough to avoid scatter of transmitted light. Coughan *et al.* concluded that the translucency of apical dentine apparently results from diminution in width of the tubules

The sclerotic apical dentine is considerably less permeable than the coronal dentine (Liden 1968). This is significant because the sclerosed dentinal tubules are less readily penetrated or are impenetrable by microorganisms or other irrigants.

APICAL PULP TISSUE

The apical pulp tissue is structurally different from the coronal pulp tissue. It consists of mainly cellular connective tissue and few collagen fibres; the apical pulp tissue is also more fibrous and contains fewer cells. Histochemically, larger concentrations of glycogen are present in the apical pulp tissue (Russell, 1967; Yamasaki *et al.*, 1986), a condition similar to the presence of an anaerobic environment. The bovine root pulp cells contain latent collagenase and a potent collagenase inhibitor (Kishi and Hayakawa, 1985). The inhibitor found to be 10 times greater in the pulp than in the coronal pulp (Kishi *et al.*, 1985). The reasons for this difference are unknown. In addition, higher concentration of sulphated glycosaminoglycans is present the apical pulp tissue than that present in the central pulp tissue (Zerosi, 1967). The exact significance of these findings is not yet clear.

The fibrous tissue of the apical root canal is similar to that of the periodontal ligament. The collagenous apical tissue is whitish in appearance. This fibrous structure appears as a barrier against the apical progression of pulpal inflammation. However, in partial or total pulpitis, there is no complete inhibition of inflammation of the periapical tissue. Although the apical pulp tissue is free of such exudates, inflammatory exudates may be found in the periapical tissues.

CEMENTUM

Although often missing to the apical third of the root, acellular cementum may cover the root dentine from the CEJ to the apex. Here the cementum may be entirely of the cellular type. It is thinnest at the CEJ (20–50 μm) and

19

thickest towards the apex. The AF is surrounded by the cementum. Sometimes the cementum extends to the inner wall of the dentine for short distance, thereby forming a lining of the root canal.

The term *acellular cementum* is inappropriate. As a living tissue, a cell is always an integral part of cementum However, some layers of cementum do not incorporate cells, the spider-like cementocytes, whereas other layers do contain such cells in their lacunae. Layers of cellular and acellular cementum may follow any pattern. Acellular cementum can at times be found on the surface of cellular cementum. Cellular cementum is frequently formed at the surface of acellular cementum, but it may compromise the entire thickness of the apical cementum. It is invariably thickest around the apex and, by its growth, contributes to the length of the root.

The thickness of cementum reflects one of its functions. It is about 20–50 µm at the cementoenamel junction and 20–150 µm in the apical third of the root. The thickness of cementum is greater at the apex because continuous deposition of cementum during the eruptive phase of the tooth to preserve its height in the occlusal plane. The continuous deposition of cementum is also responsible for forming the mature AF. As it matures, the foramen becomes conical, with the apex of the cone, called the minor diameter, facing the pulp and the base, called the major diameter, facing the periodontal ligament. The continuous deposition of cementum also increases the major diameter and results in an average 0.2–0.5 mm deviation of the AF from the centre of the root apex. Although CDJ may coincide with the minor diameter, cementum may grow unevenly and may change this relationship.

One of the major functions of the cementum is repair. Root fractures and resorptions are usually repaired by cementum. The closing of the immature roots by apexification procedures is done by deposition of cementum-like tissue. Cementum also has protective function. Probably because of its vascularity, cementum is more resistant to resorption than bone. Consequently, orthodontic movement of roots can usually be performed with a minimum of resorptive damage. Other functions of cementum include the maintenance of the periodontal width by continuous deposition and the sealing of the accessory and apical foramina after root canal therapy.

Hypertrophy or Hyperplasia of Cementum

The term *hyperplasia* is used when in case there is an over growth of cementum in response to the function. Under abnormal stress, the periodontal fibres and/or cementum may be torn, or a spike-like hypercementosis may develop. When only the periodontal fibres are torn, the cementum in which the torn fibres are embedded is resorbed. New fibres are then formed and new cementum is deposited in the resorbed area. When heavy stress is placed on a tooth, a thickened amount of cementum is deposited, thereby increasing the area of periodontal attachment and strengthening the supporting mechanism. This increased deposition of cementum with regard to function is called hypertrophy or hypercementosis.

When an overgrowth of cementum occurs for no apparent reason, it is called hyperplasia. Excessive amount of cementum is present in both instances. Difficulties in extraction are created by the presence of hyperplastic cementum. In endodontic therapy, instrumentation and filling of root canal would then be performed considerably short of radiographic apex.

Hyperplasia of cementum is also thought to be a response to the presence of infection or inflammation of the apical tissue (Boyle, 1960). If a periapical granuloma is untreated for a long time, it may cause such an overgrowth or hyperplasia of cementum that a root end assumes a knob-like appearance. This type of response is indicative of a favourable prognosis for

21

endodontic therapy. In favourable conditions, instead of an overgrowth of cementum, resorption of cementum and dentine may occur.

Cementum is usually more resistant to resorptive process than bone possibly because it is without blood supply. Only the surface of the cementum is in contact with the blood vessels from the periodontal ligament.

PERIODONTAL LIGAMENT

The periodontal ligament is a dense, fibrous tissue that supports and attaches the tooth to its socket. It is widest at the bony crest and narrowest just below the centre of the root and widens again in the apical region.

Periodontal ligament fibres are divided into five groups, among which the apical fibre group revolves around the apical part of the tooth. Oxytalan fibres are distributed throughout the periodontal ligament, but they are numerous in the transeptal region. At the apex of the tooth, oxytalan fibres form a complex network and run in many directions.

The exact role of the oxytalan fibre system is unclear. The assigned roles include additional mechanical strength, guidance of incisor tooth eruption, maintenance of vascular stability and patency, and participation of the mechanism of proprioception related to vascular flow.

VASCULAR AND NEURAL SUPPLY THROUGH

THE APICAL THIRD

The neurovascular bundle enters the pulp through the apical foramina. It consists of one or two arterioles with their sympathetic nerve fibres and myelinated and unmyelinated sensory nerves entering the pulp, and two or three venules and lymphatic vessels exiting the pulp. Accessory foramina may serve as portals of entry and exit from the blood vessels in some teeth.

The fibrous structure of the apical pulp tissue supports the blood vessels and nerves entering the pulp. The pulp of the tooth is supplied by many blood vessels originating in the medullary space of the bone surrounding the root apex. The blood vessels run between the bone trabeculae and through the periodontal ligament before entering the apical foramina as arteries or arterioles. However, occasionally the width of the entering vessels ramifies in the apical pulp tissue. The micro angiographs reveal that on entering the AF, the apical artery divides immediately into several principal or central arteries (de Saunders, 1967). The blood vessels are surrounded by large medullated nerves, which also branch after they enter the pulp. As the blood vessels approach the centre of the pulp, they branch and become wider.

The close relationship of the blood and nerve supplies of the pulp and periodontal ligament provides a background for interrelationship of pulp and periodontal disease. An inflammatory or degenerative process involving periodontal ligament could affect its blood supply and that of some portions of the pulp. Conversely, a disease process affecting the pulpal blood vessel would probably affect some of the blood vessels of the periodontal ligament. As the nerve supply likewise is similar for both the pulp and the periodontal ligaments, periodontal inflammation may cause pain similar to a toothache caused by pulpitis.

Chapter 4

REASON FOR ROOT CURVATURE

When the tooth erupts into the oral cavity and becomes functional, its root formation is not completed. It is wide open and the Hertwig's epithelial root sheath (HERS), a circular curtain like structure, is active with its root formative function.

Two important things may happen as this tooth becomes functional It is made to bear the biting stress that may push it in the mesial direction and The occlusal load may disturb the HERS at the apical third.

The reason for the abundant occurrence of accessory canals and curvature in the apical third may be a break in the continuity of the circular curtain-like structure of the root sheath, because of the stress transmitted by the biting forces.

BULL'S EYE APPEARANCE

Frequently, root formation brings about severe curvature. When the curvature is to the mesial or distal, which is frequently seen in maxillary lateral incisors or occasionally premolars, there is little problem in detecting it. However, when it is to the buccal or lingual (in the direction of the central X-ray beam), it is more difficult to detect the curvature. Upon close scrutiny, it may show an increased radiopacity at the end of root where the root doubles back on itself and is actually "X-rayed" twice. In extreme cases, a peculiar *target* or *bull's* appearance is present in the film.

MAXILLARY CENTRAL INCISOR

From the labiolingual point of view, the pulp canal space tapers evenly from the cervical line where it is triangular in cross section to the apical foramen where it has a circular cross-sectional configuration. From both a labiolingual and mesiodistal viewpoints, the shape of the canal is conical and relatively straight with a blunted rounded apex. The shape of the cross-sectional area in the apical portion is circular to ovoid.

The mean distance of the apical foramen to the root apex ranges from 0.30 to 0.49 mm. The apical foramen is found within 1 mm of the root apex. The frequency of occurrence of lateral canals is high in this tooth, probably the highest among all the teeth. Interestingly, the canals do not seem to exit randomly but have propensity to exit on the labial or mesial surface of the root. The root apex of the central incisor is placed labially, closely approximating the external cortical plate that facilitates surgical access to the root.

MAXILLARY LATERAL INCISOR

In maxillary lateral incisor, the root is slender, which is wider labiolingually than mesiodistally. The root apex is relatively sharper than that of central incisor, showing a common deflection to the distal and palatal. Therefore, although the canal may seem to exit at the radiographic apex and anatomically it dose exit within 0.5 mm of the apex, the direction of its exit proceeds distalpalatally.

The apical portion of the lateral incisor is palatally placed from the labial cortical plate, located centrally or distal palatally in the

cancellous portion of the alveolar bone[19]. The percentage of success after endodontic therapy of these teeth is not as favourable as that of central

25

incisor. The probable reasons are unpredictability of the morphology at the apical third, it frequently shows curvatures distally or palatally, and the possibility of developmental anomalies[6].

MAXILLARY CANINE

The root of this tooth is wider labial-lingually than that of incisors. The ridiculer pulp space is also much wider in the dimension in the coronal and middle third. In the apical third, the canal becomes constricted mesiodistally. The canal is usually an even narrow canal that tapers to the single foramen. Cross-sectionally, the mid root is ovoid, which gradually becomes circular in the apical third.

The canine root is normally straight, single, and symmetrical labial-lingually as it tapers to relatively sharp apex. However, rare incidence of bifidity has been reported. The root is bent distal to the crown and, in addition to this slight divergence of coronal and radicular axes, the apical part of the root is often more abruptly curved distally, sometimes labiodistally. From a mesial/distal aspect, the root is much wider with a slight convexity cervical-apically on both labial and lingual margins, whereas the central portion of the proximal surface is usually flattened or concave. The mean distance of the apical foramen from the root apex ranges from 0.30 to 0.62 mm.

MAXILLARY FIRST PREMOLAR

Maxillary first premolar usually have two roots. Single canal may be found in 10% teeth. According to a study carried out by Carns and Skidmore, it was found in 3 in 6% of the

26

Teeth. Tooth shows a combination of root canal systems type I–IV, as described by Weine. When the variations in the root canal system are present, there is an increased likelihood of anastomosis throughout the length of the canals.

The tooth length ranges from 22.5 to 23.5 mm with the apical foramina being at a mean distance of 0.55 mm from the anatomic apex. The canal outline is similar to the canine with the mid root, and the shape of the apical cross sections is generally round. All root surfaces are convex taper to apices that are sharp in cross section at the mid to apical root level. Both roots are approximately round with buccal root outline slightly greater in circumference.

Coupled with the divergent roots of the first premolar, a fenestration of the apical third of the buccal root is common. Surgical reduction of the apex in to the bony housing of the alveolar process is often necessary for healing of the radicular bone. The apical third of the root requires due consideration. It may be very thin and frequently show a distal curvature. Forceful instrumentation may cause due errors. Hence, procedurally, the apical third should be treated cautiously. Apical foramen is generally close to the radiographic apex.

MAXILLARY SECOND PREMOLAR

Maxillary second premolars are mostly single rooted. The number of canals according to vertucci is the following: 75% one canal, 24% two canals, 1% three canals[3]. Morphologically, this tooth is complicated. Morfis*et al.* after studying morphology of the apical foramen under scanning electron microscope concluded that second premolar has the most complicated apical morphologic make up of all the teeth. Maxillary second premolars commonly show the following morphological features that are of clinical significance:

1. This tooth is unique compared to other teeth in the location of apical foramen. When it is single-rooted, the foramen may be found 0.9–1.8 mm short of the radiographic apex. Therefore, whenever working length is determined, it is important to take necessary care.

2. Compared to other teeth, the frequency of occurrence of multiple foramina is quite high in the maxillary second premolar. The main canal may split in the apical part of the root into few before exiting separately.

Chapter 5

Age Change at Apex

Ageing of the individual is manifested at all levels – from the macromolecular to that of population. Age-related changes are considered to be a result of biological activities and are associated with minor disturbances.

Ageing can also be defined as the combination of process beyond development and maturation that results in a diminution of capacity of the tissues.

GENERAL EFFECTS OF AGEING

Ageing is manifested to different degree and in different manners at various times, but in all tissues it includes general features such as:

1. Tissue dessication

2. Decrease cellular component

3. Reduce number and quality of blood vessel and nerve

4. Increase number and thickness of collegen fibre

5. Diminished size of pulp

CHANGE IN APICAL DENTINE

o   Odntoblasts appear to undergo degeneration and atrophy

o   Increased peritublar dentine or increased deposition of crystal leads to occlusion of dentinal tubule. This condition is called sclerosis of dentine. Sclerosis of dentine in the apical third occurs consistently with age.

o Secondary dentine is deposited continuously by the radicluar pulp tissue. It is seen on the root canal walls of some teeth and in greater quantities in teeth involved periodontally.

o Sclerosis reduces permeability of dentine and may help prolong pulp vitality.

o Mineral density is greater in this area, as shown by radiography and permeability studies.

o Appear transparent or light in transmitted light and dark in reflected light.

o The decrease in the number of odontoblasts is paralleled by loss of cells, inducing fibroblasts, in the pulp proper of old teeth.

This variable structure which is situated in the apical region presents challenges for root canal therapy. Successful sealing in the apical region may not be provided by obturation techniques that rely on the penetration of adhesives into dentinal tubules. Conversely, the decrease in dentinal tubules present in this apical region leads to decreased chances of bacterial invasion into the dentinal walls of the root.

AGE-RELATED CHANGES IN APICAL PULP

- Reduction in size and volume of the pulp.

- The basic reduction in the coronal pulp areas is the result of a continual apposition of dentine occlusally as well at furcation area.

- Deposition of dentine at furcation area is greater than that of occlusal dentine.

- Secondary dentine formation occurs continuously throughout life and may finally result in complete pulp eradication. In maxillary anterior teeth, the secondary dentine is formed on the lingual of the pulp chamber; in molar teeth the max deposition occurs on the floor of the chamber.

Denticles are formed around foci of mineralizing pulp tissue components such as collagen and nerve fibres, blood vessels, ground substance, and inflamed and necrotic cells. They are composed of tubular dentine and a tubular mineralized material, and because they are partially or completely surrounded by dentine, they can be attached or embedded. Approximately 15% of teeth show pulp stone in the apical third of the root, and more than one pulp stone is often found.

There may be some difficulties in root canal instrumentation because of the presence of denticles within the pulp tissue in the apical third of the root. They may become detached and impacted into the apical foramen during reaming or filing of root canal, rendering further instrumentation difficult.

Clinical Features

- Is a common feature in teeth of individuals aged more than 45 years.

- Located in root pulp or coronal pulp or both.

- They are generally first seen in root pulp of isolated calcified masses. In other teeth, multiple larger masses are observed, which may apparently obliterate the root canal.

- Isolated masses coalesce to form large mass that fuse with dentine.

31

- The calcified masses in the apical pulp are smaller and merge to obliterate the normal pulp architecture.

- There is a direct link of these masses with the collagen fibres.

- Milch postulated that with increased cross-linkage of collagen in apical area during advancing age there is an enhanced tendency among these fibres to become mineralized.

Decrease in Number of Cells

- The number of cells is found to be reduced by 50% in aged pulps.

- Fibroblasts show degeneration with advancing age, as represented by small size and a reduced number of organelles, including RER, mitochondria, and Golgi complex.

- Increase in the number of vacuoles and gradual degenerative changes lead to absence of cells over some or all the pulpal surface.

- One of the first changes to be observed to the small arteries in the root pulp in ageing teeth is osteosclerotic change.

- The intima of the vessel becomes thick, resulting in small lumen.

- The old blood capillaries show a widening of the basement membranes with strongly periodic acid-Schiff-positive staining whereas the young vessels appear to have thin lightly red stained membrane.

- In the diffuse calcification process of the root pulp, the adventitia and media of the small arteries and veins as well as the walls of the capillaries become mineralized, which leads to loss of vessels in the old pulps.

- As with blood vascular system, the nerves within the root pulp show changes as a result of the diffuse calcification. The connective tissue (CT) sheath of the nerve bundles becomes mineralized. The paucity of nerves in old pulps is seen cuspal nerves and their terminal branching is absent. Nerve fibres that persist show degeneration such as reticulation, fragmentation, and beading.

- Capillary permeability decreases with age, and transfer of substances from blood to cells may be shown during ageing.

Changes in Collagenous Elements

- Increase in collagenous elements of the pulp during the ageing process.

- Apical pulps of old teeth show a relative decrease in the number of thick collagenous bundles compare to coronal.

- The prominence of fibre bundles in old pulps may be, in part, attributed to the persistence of the CT sheaths in a narrowed pulpal chamber after the vascular and neural structures are decreased or lost.

Von Korff Fibres

- During the ageing process, the Von Korff fibres (collagenous fibres that emerge from the predentin and pass into the pulp) become accentuated.

33

Changes in Ground Substance

- The presence of calcified masses in the root pulp accentuates the Schiff intensity, becoming red.

- When there is diffuse calcification in the apical pulp, the calcified masses stain Schiff positive in contrast to the surrounding pulpal ground substance that appear deep blue.

- Bhussrey and Zerlotti reported a decrease in muco polysaccharides in ageing pulps, and that the amount of amorphous ground substances decreases as the number of collagen fibrils increases in skin and elsewhere.

Vascular and Nerve Distribution

- Ageing leads to degranulative changes to vascular and nerve supply to pulp. In root pulps of old teeth, there is narrowing of the circumference.

CEMENTUM AT APEX

- Cementum is about 20–50μm thick at CEJ and 20–150μm thick at the apicalthird of the root.

- The greater thickness of cementum at the apex is due to continuous deposition during the eruptive phase of tooth, and to preserve its height in the occlusal plane.

- Owing to ageing, the smooth surface of the cementum becomes rough due to calcification of some bundles of ligament fibres at the place of their attachment to cementum.

- This happens on all cemental surfaces except in the apical area. In the apical area, due to ageing, continuous cementum deposition occurs, which sometimes may lead to closure of apical foramen.

- Owing to ageing, sometimes cementum deposition can also occur, creating reversal lines.

MANAGEMENT OF CALCIFIED CANALS

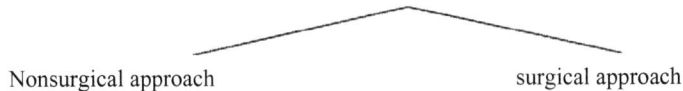

Nonsurgical approach   surgical approach

NONSURGICAL APPROACH

Nonsurgical management is the first-line treatment of calcified canals. The important considerations in this approach are as follows:

- Recognition of the orifice

- Biomechanical preparation of a calcified canal

- Role of chelating agent

- When to stop looking?

- Complications

These are evaluated in detail subsequently.

RECOGNITION OF THE ORIFICE

A practitioner first mentally visualizes and projects the normal spatial relationship of the pulp space onto anX-ray of the calcified tooth in order to locate the calcified orifice. Then the two-dimensional radiographic image is correlated with the three-dimensional morphology of the tooth. It is important to remember that the canal space in normal root canal anatomy is always in the cross-sectional centre of the root. Similarly, the pulp chamber is (or was, before calcification) located in the cross-sectional centre of the crown.[5]

In a tooth with a calcified pulp chamber, the distance from the occlusal/incisal surface to the projected pulp chamber is measured from a preoperative periradicular film, or preferably from a bite-wing film, which enhances accuracy.

It is helpful to locate the orifice before placing the rubber dam. This helps a dentist to evaluate the relationships of root and work more effectively in the long axis of the tooth. However, the dental dam must be placed before proceeding further once the canal is located.

Khabbaz and Serefoglou found the use of two working radiographs to locate calcified canals (as proposed by Walton) inadequate. They found this method to be useful only in cases where the head of the bur and the canal had enough distance between them. When they are closed together, as in most cases, a third radiograph is obligatory to give the third dimension of the root. For the determination of calcified root canals, the authors applied the buccal object rule, which is as follows:

After the initial access opening, the bur is left in place and three radiographs are taken:

- Straight on to the buccolingual dimension in order to determine theposition of the head ofthe bur in the root canal in the mesiodistal dimension.

- With a 20°*horizontal angulation* with the cone shifted *distally*.

- With a 20°*horizontal angulation* with the cone directed *mesially*.

The last two X-rays give information about the relation of the bur with the canal lumen in the buccolingual dimension.

BIOMECHANICAL PREPARATION OF A CALCIFIED CANAL

Coronal flaring in a crown-down manner is preferred. In some cases, incremental instrumentation makes it possible to place instrument without forcing, and the correct working length is achieved without the use of forceful reaming action. With the step or flared preparation, the smaller and more flexible files are used to the full potential; however the larger and more rigid instruments are put away from the apex and restricted to the straighter portions of the canal, where they do not significantly change the original shape of the canal.

Incremental instrumentation is attained by constructing new increments between the established widths by cutting off a portion of the file tip, thus making its diameter slightly wider. For example, if a 1-mm segment is clipped from a size 10 file, the instrument becomes a size 12. By trimming sizes 15, 20, and 25, instruments of sizes 17, 22, and 27, respectively, can be created. In extremely sclerotic canals, only 0.5 mm segments are trimmed, which increases the width of the instrument by 0.01mm and transform a size 10 into a size 11, etc. because cutting the shaft yields a flat tip, a metal nail file is used to smoothen the end and re-establish a bevel after the removal of any segment.[15]

ROLE OF CHELATING AGENT

Chelator preparations have been encouraged frequently as adjuncts for root canal preparation, especially in narrow and calcified root canals. However, to what extent these agents actually facilitate negotiation and preparation of such canals is unknown. This is because of not only the difficulty in providing a sufficient amount of chelator to this part of the root canal, but also the differences in structure between the middle, coronal, and apical dentines. Apical dentine is more frequently sclerosed and is more mineralized. To identify the entrance to calcified canals, the authors recommend that liquid EDTA solution should be introduced into the pulp chamber (pipette, cotton pellet).

WHEN TO STOP LOOKING?

COMPLICATIONS

SURGICAL APPROACH

The teeth must be treated with periradicular surgery in cases of calcific metamorphosis, if the teeth are symptomatic, or in cases where the canal cannot be negotiated. When compared with perforations and root fractures, retrograde procedures become more conservative. Currently advocated techniques of preparing a concave root face, followed by a dentine bonding agent and resin composite root-end fill, seem promising and may solve the issue of contaminated tissue debris at the resected root end.[1] If periradicular surgery fails and symptoms are still there, the only option remaining is the extraction of the concerned tooth.

Chapter 6

Pathology of the Apex

The term *apical periodontitis* is generally used to describe and group together the various periapical conditions that arise from pulp disease but there are many different pathological conditions that fall under this group of disorders.

CLASSIFICATIONS OF PERIAPICAL DISEASES

Apical periodontitis has been classified into the following five categories by the WHO:

6. Acute apical periodontitis of pulpal origin

7. Chronic apical periodontitis of pulpal origin

8. Periapical abscess with sinus

9. Periapical abscess without sinus

10. Radicular cysts

As this classification does not include the structural aspects of periapical lesions, an alternative classification, which was based on the histopathology and dynamics of these lesions with strict criteria to define each entity, was proposed byNair(1997) .

We can summarize Nair's classification of periapicalradiolucencies as follows:

o Clinically normal periapical/periradicular tissues

o Apical periodontitis

      Acute: Primary

Secondary (or acute exacerbation)

Chronic: Granuloma

Condensing osteitis

3. Periapical cyst

    a. True cyst

    b. Pocket cyst

4. Periapical abscess

    a. Acute: Primary

        Secondary

    b. Chronic

5. Facial cellulitis

6. Extra-radicular infection

7. Foreign body reaction

8. Periapical scar

9. Apical root resorption

    a. Inflammatory

    b. Replacement

    c. Pressure

    d. Orthodontic

    e. Physiological

It is to be remembered that these terms do not account for the different pathological entities that occur during the progression of peri apical disease through its various stages. Each stage of peri apical disease should be considered as part of a continuum of stages that occur during the development and progression of the disease processes.

Moreover, peri apical diseases are usually a result of pulp disease and hence the signs and symptoms of peri apical disease will be present in conjunction with the signs and symptoms of the concurrent pulp disease.

PRIMARY APICAL PERIODONTITIS

Pathogenesis

The initial periapical response to bacterial presence within the canal or to bacterial invasion of the periapical region will be an acute inflammatory response, known as primary acute apical periodontitis.

Such a reaction may also be caused by trauma or by endodontic instrumentation procedures and irritant materials. Primary acute apical periodontitis, which is usually of short duration, occurs within a previously healthy periapical region.

Clinical Symptoms

- Teeth having primary acute apical periodontitis have very significant tenderness to percussion and pain when there is pressure on the tooth.

- The tooth may have increased mobility, and the pain normally occurs suddenly and unexpectedly. .

- The patient will be aware of considerable pain, soreness to biting and on touching the tooth, and possibly a feeling of pressure buildingup in the periapical region.

Radiographic Features

Looking radiographically, the periodontal ligament space and lamina dura may look normal or there may appear as a slight thickening of the periodontal ligament space and some loss of the lamina dura around the apex of the tooth root.

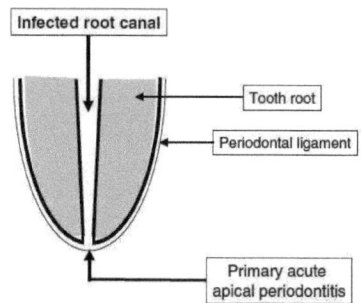

Primary Acute Apical Periodontitis

Figure 1: Diagrammatic representation of the radiographic finding of primary acute apical periodontitis. Though there appears a periapical inflammatory response, it is not yet confirmed radiographically if there is no bone or root resorption to create a widening of the periodontal ligament space or radiolucency. (Note: other conditions appearing similar include primary acute apical abscess and facial cellulitis associated with a primary abscess.)

SECONDARY APICAL PERIODONTITIS

Pathogenesis

Secondary acute apical periodontitis is an acute exacerbation of a pre-existing chronic apical periodontitis lesion. This may occur in the form of an abscess (secondary apical abscess) when bacteria move out of the root canal and infect the periapical tissues, although other local or systemic changes may also be responsible for an acute exacerbation of the inflammation.

Clinical Symptoms

A patient having secondary acute apical periodontitis experiences similar pain symptoms to those present in primary acute apical periodontitis but it is possible to find many clinical and radiographic signs present to assist the diagnosis as it is an acute exacerbation of an established chronic apical periodontitis lesion.

- There may be a history of episodes of pain or discomfort but many patients may not remember them..

Radiological Feature

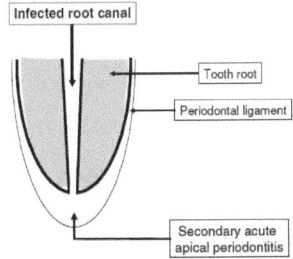

Infected root canal

Tooth root

Periodontal ligament

Secondary acute apical periodontitis

Secondary Acute Apical Periodontitis

Figure 2: Diagrammatic representation of the radiographic appearance of secondary acute apical periodontitis. (Note: other conditions that may appear similar are the following: secondary acute apical abscess, facial cellulitis associated with a secondary abscess, extra-radicular infection, chronic apical periodontitis, periapical granuloma, chronic apical abscess, periapical scars, and periapical cysts – pocket and true.)

Radiographically, there appears a radiolucency surrounding the apex of the involved tooth and also a loss of the lamina dura. The size of the radiolucency depends primarily on how long the chronic apical periodontitis is persisting – it may be just a widened periodontal ligament space in early cases to even a large radiolucent area present for long. However, these lesions progress at varying rates so the size of the area does not necessarily indicate the time it has been present.

CHRONIC APICAL PERIODONTITIS

Pathogenesis

If no treatment is started, then there will be persistence of irritants in the apical part of the root canal system. Then, the initial acute inflammation slowly changes to a chronic inflammatory reaction, histologically known as a periapical granuloma.

Clinical Symptoms

- Chronic apical periodontitis can differ in its clinical presentation as this general term represents different histological conditions of the periapical disease process.

- Usually patients are unaware of any symptoms associated with these lesions, which are frequently noted as incidental findings when a routine radiographic examination is conducted.

- The pulp will be necrotic and infected, or otherwise the root canal will be pulpless and infected, or previously root-filled and infected.

- There will be no response to pulp sensibility tests.

- The tooth is not tender to percussion, pressure, or palpation but it may feel "different" to these tests and it may be slightly mobile.

Radiological Findings

- Radiographically, there will be a radiolucency surrounding the apex of the involved tooth and there will be loss of the lamina dura.

- Chronic apical periodontitis can occasionally present as condensing osteitis (also known as idiopathic bone sclerosis). Here, periapical bone will appear more radiopaque than normal bone. Some case may also have a slightly widened periodontal ligament space between the tooth root and the radiopacity.

PERIAPICAL CYSTS

Pathogenesis

Nair has defined two types of periapical cysts: periapical pocket cysts and periapical true cysts.

A periapical pocket cyst is a sac-like epithelium-lined cavity that is open to, and continuous with, the root canal whereas the lumen of a periapical true cyst is completely enclosed by the epithelial lining and there is no communication with the root canal.

Periapical cysts are understood as a direct sequel of a periapical granuloma although not every granuloma becomes a periapical true cyst. It is not dependent on the presence or absence of irritants within the canal (as there is no contact with them) and therefore true cysts are understood to be "self-sustaining" lesions, which require to be removed surgically.

The pathway of development and the histological appearance of stratified squamous epithelial lining and the rest of the pocket cyst wall are similar to those of a true cyst. Therefore, it can be suggested, even if it is not proven yet, that a pocket cyst may detach from the root apex and the epithelial lining may completely close to form a true cyst.

Clinical Symptoms

Both periapical true cysts and periapical pocket cysts are considered to be forms of chronic apical periodontitis.

As of other chronic periapical conditions, there exist no symptoms and the clinical diagnosis is based on radiographic findings.

However, the final diagnosis of a cyst can only be made by histological examination of a biopsy including the root apex, along with comprehensive serial sectioning.

Radiological Findings

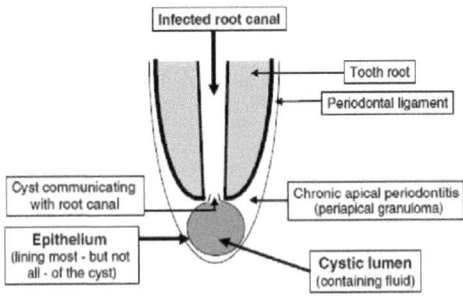

Periapical Pocket Cyst

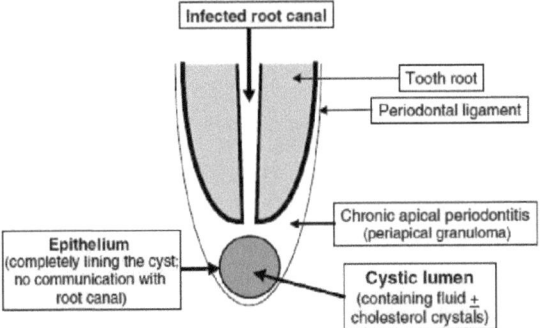

Periapical True Cyst

Periapical granulomata and radicular cysts generally have exactly the same clinical and radiographic appearance.

Only the appearance of the borders of the radiolucency cannot be used as a basis of diagnosis to distinguish between these conditions, as previously attempted by many clinicians who have incorrectly claimed that a well-defined border indicates a radicular cyst.

Now it is agreed that a well-defined border simply indicates a long-standing lesion that is gradually getting bigger whereas a diffuse border is more likely to indicate a rapidly expanding lesion.

The size of the radiolucency is also irrelevant to the histological state of the tissue as both small and large lesions can be granulomata, abscesses, or cysts.

PERIAPICAL ABSCESS

Pathogenesis

An abscess means "a localized collection of pus" and this term should be used only when there is evidence of pus formation and collection.

Apical abscesses may be either acute or chronic, and an acute apical abscess may be either a primary or a secondary lesion.

An acute abscess that grows as a result of primary acute apical periodontitis is known as a primary acute apical abscess whereas an acute abscess that develops as a result of secondary acute apical periodontitis or chronic apical periodontitis is known as a secondary acute apical abscess.

Clinical Findings

Acute periapical abscess

Both forms of acute abscess can be very painful conditions characterized by severe throbbing and pain to even light pressure, biting, touching, and percussion.

These symptoms may be accompanied by tenderness to palpation and increased mobility of the tooth.

Systemic signs of malaise, fever, and lymph node involvement may occur.

An intra-oral and/or extra-oral swelling may be present and this swelling will be fluctuant as well as tender to pressure and palpation.

The tooth involved in the abscess will have a necrotic and infected pulp, or a pulpless and infected root canal system, or it may have undergone endodontic treatment, with continued or subsequent infection of the root canal system.

Chronic apical abscess

A chronic periapical abscess is not usually associated with pain and is typically characterized by the clinical presence of a draining sinus on the oral mucosa or occasionally on the facial skin.

However, a draining sinus will be seen only when drainage occurs, and this drainage will generally occur only when pressure is built up within the periapical region.

Radiological Findings

A primary acute apical abscess may not involve any periapical changes clearly seen on a radiograph or there may be just a slight thickening of the periodontal ligament space as the periapical inflammation and fluid buildup causes extrusion of the tooth from its normal position..

A secondary acute apical abscess will have a periapical radiolucent area as it is a sequel to secondary acute apical periodontitis (which is also known as an acute exacerbation of chronic apical periodontitis).

A chronic apical abscess will have a periapical radiolucency and evidence of causative factors (e.g. caries).

FACIAL CELLULITIS

Pathogenesis

Facial cellulitis is the result of an infection when it spreads between the fascial planes because of the tissue-dissolving capacity of extra-virulent organisms.

Cellulitis may be a result of a chronic apical abscess, a primary acute apical abscess or a secondary acute apical abscess.

The spread of pus follows the pathway(s) of least resistance, which usually implies the fascial planes between the muscles of the face, head, and neck.

Spreading infections can have serious and even life-threatening consequences if not treated, and therefore, immediate and aggressive therapy is indicated.

Clinical Symptoms

Some of the features of cellulitis caused by an infected root canal system are similar to those of an acute periapical abscess (i.e. severe pain, tenderness to percussion and light touch, tooth mobility, malaise, fever, lymph node involvement, etc.) as the cellulitis is the result of an untreated or rapidly developing abscess.

However, the swelling of a cellulitis is far more severe and widespread than that ofan acute apical abscess, and it is usually less fluctuant with a "harder feel" to palpation.

The tooth causing the cellulitis will have a necrotic and infected pulp, or a pulpless and infected root canal system, or it may have had previous endodontic treatment with continued or subsequent infection of the root canal system.

Radiological Finding Radiographically, cellulitis may have a periapical radiolucency–this depends on whether it is a sequel to a primary apical abscess (no radiolucency or just a widened periodontal ligament space) or it is a sequel to a secondary apical abscess (a radiolucency will be present).

FOREIGN BODY REACTION

Aetiology

A foreign body reaction is an inflammatory response to a foreign material within the periapical tissues.

The foreign material is most likely to be excess root-filling material, such as gutta-percha or a root canal cement that has been extruded through the apical foramen during endodontic treatment.

Clinical Symptoms

The patient may show clinical symptoms such as tenderness to palpation and percussion.

In the initial stages, it is usually impossible to distinguish between a foreign body reaction and inflammation caused by an infection as a foreign body reaction can be diagnosed only with the help of a biopsy and histological examination.

Radiological Findings

Radiographically, a foreign body reaction may appear as a periapical radiolucent area surrounding radiopaque material.

Root resorption

Shallow resorption of dentin in the apical portion of the root canal isa normal occurrence. Resorption of cementum and dentin occurs on the body of the root also at the periapical region. Apical root resorption is mainly due to the following reasons:

a) rthodontic tooth movement

b) Inflammation of apical pulp and periapical periodontal tissues

Orthodontically induced root resorption is mediated by prostaglandins elaborated by localized cells that stimulate osteoblastic activity. The resorption widens the apical foramen, leaving a funnel-shaped structure. As inflammation subsides, repair of resorbed region occurs by deposition of secondary cementum.

Chapter 7

Radiographic Assessment of Apical Third

ANATOMICAL CONSIDERATIONS

Bone Structure

In the maxilla:

- the facial cortex is thin as far posterior as the disto-buccal root of the first molar. The buccal root tips are sometimes uncovered by bone.

- The buccal cortex of the second and third molars is thicker.

- The palatinal cortex of the alveolar process is thicker than that of the facial one, though it is paper-thin over the palatinal alveolus of the first molar and thinner over the palatinal alveoli of the second and third molars.

- The cancellous bone is thick over the deeper portions of the alveoli palatinal of the anterior teeth and premolars.

The apex of the lateral incisor is located in opposite to the palatinal cortical bone.

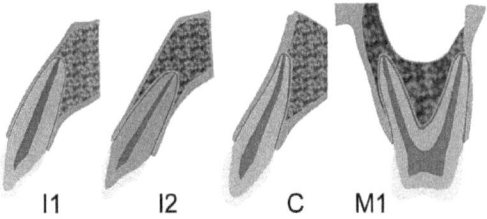

I1   I2   C   M1

Figure 1:

In the mandible:

- The alveolar process is very thin in its anterior region around the roots of incisor teeth, but it is thicker in the molar region.

- The lingual walls of the alveoli of the second and third molars are comparatively thin near the bottoms of the sockets, whereas the bone on the facial aspect is thicker and very compact. This is because of the mandible being undercut at this point for the submaxillary fossa below the mylohyoid ridge.

- The bone buccal to the last two molars is very thick, being reinforced by the external oblique ridge.

- The labial cortex surrounding the incisor apices is often thin or even absent, exposing the root tips.

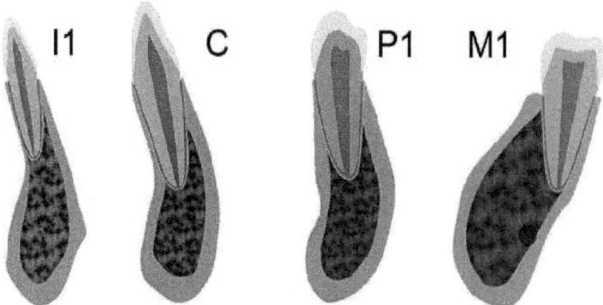

Figure 2:

Lamina Dura

The lamina dura is a continuation of the jawbone cortex, which encases the root in a socket of cortical bone. In X-rays, its appearance varies. When the X-ray beam is directed through a relatively long expanse of the structure, the lamina dura appears to be radiopaque and well defined.

However, when the beam is directed more obliquely, the lamina dura appears to be more diffuse and may not be discernible. This means that the appearance of the lamina dura depends as much on the shape and position of the root in relation to the X-ray beam as on the density and integrity of the lamina dura itself.

Besides, small differences and disruptions in the continuity of the lamina dura may be indicative of superimpositions of trabecular pattern and small nutrient canals passing from the bone to the periodontal ligament. The thickness and density of the lamina dura seen on the X-ray film may vary with the amount of occlusal stress to which the tooth is subjected.

A lesion in lamina dura may be detected on a radiograph more readily than that in a cancellous bone because more amount of mineral is removed at that site.

Although loss or diminution of the lamina dura has long been associated with a local or systemic disease, for example Paget's disease or hyperparathyroidism, there is a considerable intra- and inter-individual range in its thickness and density. Often, because the bone is frequently thin in this region, it is not possible to discern the lamina dura at the apex of the maxillary canines.

The periapical lamina dura of the other teeth may be very distinct in the same patient, Furthermore, it should be noted that some patients have a characteristically prominent well-defined lamina dura, whereas in others, it may be generally faint.

Maxillary Sinus

In one-third cases, the distance from the apices of the roots of the first molar tooth to the sinus floor is ≤ 0.5 mm. Sometimes, there is no bone between the root apex and the sinus. Therefore, a periapical X-ray may be able to show lamina dura covering the apex.

When the second molar tooth has three roots, its apices are located even closer to the maxillary sinus. The thin layer of bone covering the root can be seen as a fusion of the lamina dura and the floor of the sinus.

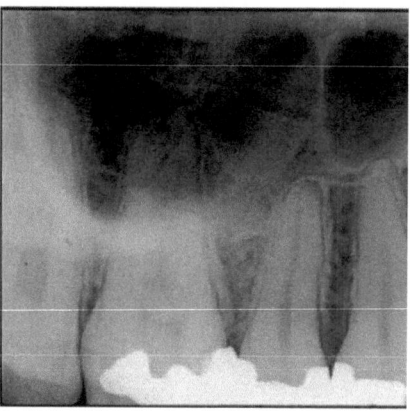

Figure 3: Septum in maxillary sinus; apparent loss of lamina dura of first molar roots.

Incisive and Mental Foramen and Mandibular Canal

The incisive foramen is the opening of the incisive canal onto the roof of the hard palate, which is located often just behind and above the roots for the central incisors.

It may pose diagnostic problems. It may appear as a radiolucent area related to the apex of the maxillary central incisors on a radiograph. Following the lamina dura or having an angled radiograph subsequently may shift the lucency in relation to apex and show its true nature.

The mental foramen opens on the facial aspect of the mandible in the region of the premolars. It may mimic periapical disease when it is projected over one of the premolar apices.

The relationship of the mandibular canal with the posterior tooth roots may differ from one in which there is close contact with all molars and the second premolar to the one in which the canal has no close relation to any posterior tooth.

When the apices of the molars are projected over the canal, the lamina dura may be overexposed, again giving the impression of missing lamina dura or a thickened periodontal ligament space that is more radiolucent than apparently normal to the patient.

Because the canal is sometimes located just below the apices of the posterior teeth, changing the vertical angle for a second film of the area does not separate the images of the apices and canal.

Visualization of Lesions in Bone

A significant distinction in the thickness of the cortices may be present in the same patient. Therefore, a lesion of a given size can be detectable in an area covered by a thin cortex; the lesion of the same size will not be seen in a region covered by thicker cortex.

Radiographic visualization of lesions is also influenced by the location of the lesions in different types of bone. The size at which the periapical lesion becomes radiologically detectable varies between the different regions of the mandible. Isolated spongiosa lesions, which are larger than 3 mm in diameter, are often easily detectable at the mandibular front teeth and premolars. Isolated spongiosa lesions at mandibular molars are often not detectable. Atypical lesions, for example discontinuities of bony structures, are particularly difficult to detect radiologically.

Frequently, the shape of the lesion is also an important factor as to whether it will be shown on the radiographs or not. For instance, an oblong lesion may not be visible on the radiographs if the exposure is at an angle through the narrowest dimension of the lesion. However, a prominent lesion might appear on the radiograph, if it is taken with the beam passing directly through the longest dimension of the lesion.

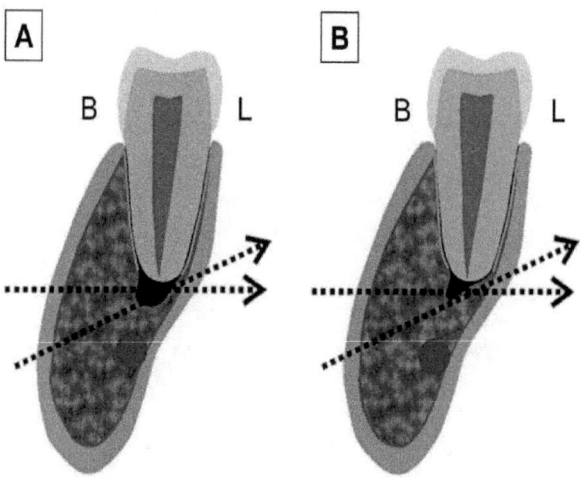

Figure 4: Effects of beam angulation and lesion size on appearance of lesion in radiographs. (A) The larger lesion in is visible from different angles. (B) The smaller and more buccally oriented lesion disappears when the beam is from an oblique angle.

PATHOLOGICAL CONSIDERATION

Periodontal Ligament

It serves as the starting point for resorptive processes and an end-point of healing processes. Periodontal membrane is more than double in width, and the presence of moderate or severe inflammation cannot be ruled out.

59

The width of periodontal ligament space may vary from patient to patient, from tooth to tooth, and even from location to location around one tooth.

A large periodontal space may be present in teeth with increased mobility due to marginal periodontitis or bruxism, but in the case of apical periodontitis, widened periodontal space is confined to the infected area near the apex.

Lamina Dura

Changes to the radiographic integrity of the lamina dura may show early evidence of the development of periapical lesion, and a radiographically visible collar-shaped increase in the thickness of the lamina dura lateral to the root may be found more often in cases with moderate-to-severe inflammation than in those with no or mild inflammation. Unfortunately, normal variations in thickness and continuity of lamina dura make the diagnosis by this criterion uncertain.

The lamina dura may be defined as irregular, indistinct, or serrate, but in the early or healing phases of apical periodontitis, none of these changes is pathognomonic. In fact, characteristics of the lamina dura may be of little help in distinguishing stages or degrees of inflammation.

Cancellous Bone

A less functionally oriented pattern replaces the normal trabecular pattern of cancellous bone if there is a root canal infection. It is easy to diagnose when mineral loss is evident. The radiolucency may be seen clearly adjacent to the root apex but may blend with the surrounding bone at the periphery of the lesion. The structure of the bone peripheral to the lamina dura or apical radiolucency may be rarefied, indicating moderate or severe inflammation.

Cortical Bone

It is easy to detect lesions in cortical bone and they assume prominence because of their clarity and size in radiographs. Root tips, and perhaps most periodontitic lesions, lie in close opposition to either the facial or the oral cortical plate.

Adjacent Structures: Maxillary Sinus and Nasal Cavity

Occasionally, the apical periodontal lesion may involve the maxillary sinus or nasal cavity and result in displacement of the floor or wall of the cavity. Odontogenic maxillary sinusitis may also be caused by periapical inflammation.

Often, the destruction, by localized inflammation, of the extremely thin bone lamella present between the sinus floor and the root apex can cause a local mucous membrane reaction in the form of membrane swellings, pseudocysts or, sometimes, chronic maxillary sinusitis.

Healing

Healing after endodontic therapy is determined by interpreting the periodic recall radiographs. A transient increase in radiolucency may be present, which may be due to chemical and/or mechanical irritation resulting from the root canal treatment and usually revert to normal.

The area of mineral loss is gradually filled with bone and the radiographic density increases. The structure of the newly formed bone may not be normal; it is often being less organized. The contours, width, and structure of the periodontal ligament become normal.

61

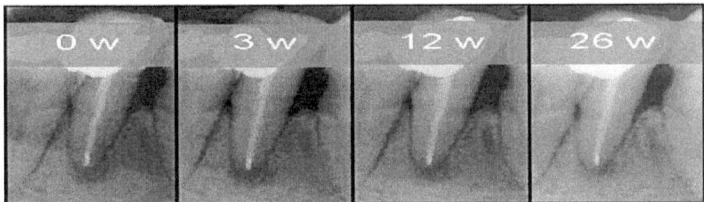

Figure 5:

PERIAPICAL SCARS

For scar tissue after surgery, the rarefaction may decrease in size and may have one or more of the following characteristics: bone structures are recognized within the rarefaction; the periphery of the rarefaction be irregular and demarcated by a compact bone border; the rarefaction is often located asymmetrically around the apex; the connection of the rarefaction with the periodontal space may be angular. Isolated scar tissue areas in the bone can be observed, but this is a later stage of healing in some cases.

APPEARANCE OF ROOT CANALS

It is not easy to identify the lateral canals, accessory canals, and other an anatomic aberrations. A clinician should have good knowledge of these anatomic variations. Clinically also, we should carefully examine for extra canals by probing the potential area using a sharp pointer or an endodontic explorer. Anatomic variations may be assessed, and sometimes identified, radiographically.

When the X-ray shows a root canal descending from the puplpal floor and suddenly stopping in the apical region, bifurcation or trifurcation in the apical region can be expected. To conform this, another radiograph is exposed from a mesial or distal angulation of 10°–

30°. This will show more roots or vertical lines, indicating peripheries of additional root surfaces.

If the shadow of root canal abruptly stops in the middle third of the root or if the diameter of the root canal suddenly narrows down, it shows that the root canal may be dividing into two. This is very common in mandibular premolars. If lateral radiolucency is present in the apical one third of the root, it may indicate lateral canal accessory canals or presence of periodontal lesions.

If a radiolucent line is running along the diagnostic instrument whose long axis is not in relation to the instrument, then there is high possibility of an additional canal. The recent advancements such as xeroradiography, radio visiography, digital substraction radiography, and computed tomography also help in identifying these minute anatomical variations.

OTHER FEATURES OF APEX ON RADIOGRAPHS

Thin "pinched" apex: Care should be taken during instrumentation to avoid perforation.

Bulbous apex: Bulbous appearance of apex is attributed to hypercementosis.Apical constriction may be significantly shorter from the radiographic apex compared to normal teeth in cases of bulbous apex.

Resorbed apex: Advanced inflammation at the periapex usually causesresorption of cementum, by widening of apical foramen. Such changes will make determination of working length difficult with proper apical

Preparation and condensation of gutta-percha. So it is recommended that apical stop should be created in such teeth.

Blunderbuss apex: A newly formed tooth generally shows anincompletely forced root having a wide root canal and an open apex. Such a canal is termed immature or blunderbuss canal.

PERIAPICAL INDEX

Periapical index (PAI) provides an ordinal scale of five scores ranging from "healthy" to "severe periodontitis with exacerbating features."

The PAI is based on reference radiographs with verified histological diagnosesoriginally published by Brynolf.

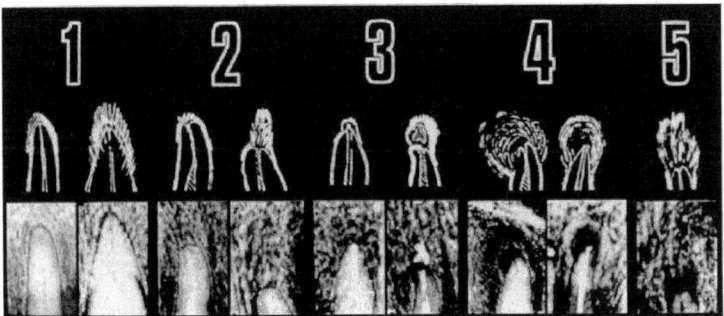

Figure 6:

1. . Normal periapical structures

2. Small changes in bone structure

3. Changes in bone structure with some mineral loss

4. Periodontitis with well-defined radiolucent area

5. Severe periodontitis with exacerbating features

Chapter8

Clinical Consideration

WORKINGLENGTH

Ingle (1973) andFrank*etal.* **(1988)** recommend working length to be 0.5–1mmfromradiographicapex.

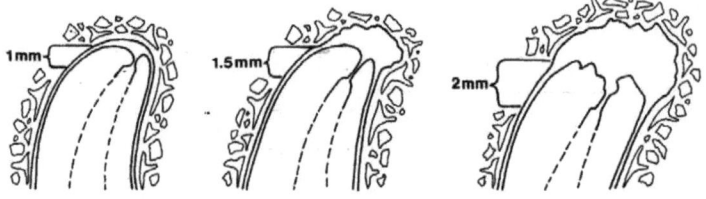

Weine*etal.* **(1996)** recommended the working length to be:

- 1 mm from apex when no root/bone resorption

- 1.5 mm from apex when only bone resorption

- 2mm from apex when both root & bone resorption

Wu*etal.* **(2000)** recommend0–3 mm working length for termination of the procedure, depending on pulpal diagnosis:

VitalCases:2–3 mm short of radiographic apex

PulpNecrosis:2 mm short of radiographic apex

RetreatmentCases:1–2 mm short of radiographic apex

For vital cases, clinical and biological evidence indicate that the ideal point at which the procedure should be terminated is 2–3 mm short of the radiographic apex .This leaves an apical pulp stump, which prevents extrusion firritating filling materials into the periradicular tissues. Bya suitable treatment,the vitality of the residual pulp may be preserved in the majority of cases, resulting in a normal apical periodontal ligament and fibrous connective tissue in the apical portion of the root canal.

With pulp necrosis, bacteria and their by-products may be present in the apical root canal, which could affect healing. Microorganisms present at the apical part of the canal have better accessibility to periapical tissue. This would allow them to get nutrition and exert harmful effects on the surrounding structure. The apicalpartsofinfectedrootcanalsshowingperiapicallesionswillaccommodat eabundantbacteria.Bacteriahavebeendetectedattheapicalforamen (AF) and found in parts inaccessible to instrumentation. Hence, it is recommended that thewholerootcanalbedisinfectedtothelevelofthe AF becausebacteriacancolo nizetheentirecanalandthrive, especially apically.

WORKINGWIDTH

Horizontaldimensionsoftherootcanalsystematworkinglengtharete rmedasworkingwidth (WW). Bystudying the cross section so fapical canals, it can be understood in a better way. Most of the canal sare of oval shape in the crosssection. They have *two* diameters –a minor (smaller) diameter and a major (larger) diameter. The cleaning quality depends on instrumenting to the larger diameter.

Chapter 9

APICAL SURGERY

The major cause of periapical lesions is a leaky apical seal permitting the egress of microorganism and other toxins. Periradicular curettage only helps to eliminate only the effect of the leakage but not the cause. Periradicular curettage alone (without apical resection) will invite the resection of the lesion. Hence, apical surgery, entails not only the removal of the diseased tissue or the root tip, but also, most importantly, the retrofilling and resealing of the root canal system. If it was possible for the entire root canal system to be cleaned and totally sealed every time, then the endodontic surgery would not be required at all. In fact, however, the complexity of the root canal system, especially in the apical region, will not permit 100% success for nonsurgical endodontic therapy. Therefore, when such failures are treated surgically, periradicular curettage must be followed by a root-end retrograde sealing with a biocompatible material.

Classification of endodontic microsurgical cases

As the endodontic surgery outcome depends on the preexisting tooth condition, the probability of success depends on the situation at hand. Therefore, we propose the following classification (Figure 1):

- *Class A*: It represents the absence of a periapical lesion, no mobility, a normal pocket depth, and unresolved symptoms after nonsurgical approaches have been exhausted. The only reason for the surgery is clinical symptoms.

- *Class B*: It represents the presence of a small periapical lesion along with clinical symptoms, normal periodontal probing depth, and no mobility. The ideal candidates for microsurgery are the teeth that lie in this class.

- *Class C*: It represents the presence of a large periapical lesion progressing coronally without having periodontal pocket and no mobility.

- *Class D*: It represents the teeth that are clinically similar to those of Class C but have deep periodontal pockets.

- *Class E*: It represents the presence of a deep periapical lesion with an endodontic–periodontal communication to the apex but no obvious fracture.

- *Class F*: It represents the presence of an apical lesion and complete denudement of the buccal plate and no mobility.

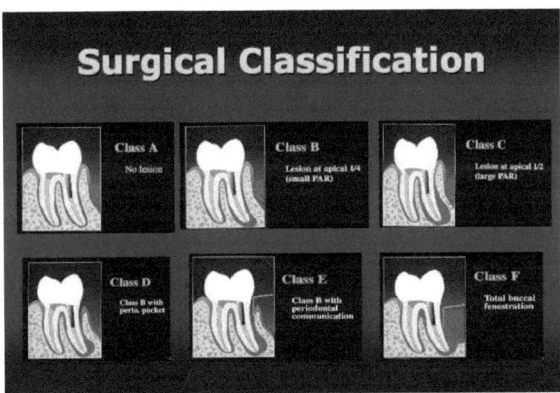

Figure 1:

Extent of resection

The extent of root resection does not completely satisfy biological principles. Gilheany et al. suggest that at least 2 mm should be removed for minimizing bacterial leakage from the canals. The anatomical study of the root apex shows that at least 3 mm root-end must be removed to reduce 98% apical ramifications and 93% lateral canals. As these percentages are very similar at 4 mm from the apex, root-end amputation of 3 mm is recommended, because this leaves on an average of 7–9 mm of the root, which provides sufficient strength and stability. A root-end amputation of less than 3mm is unlikely to remove all of the lateral canals and apical ramifications, hence posing a risk of reinfection and eventual failure.

Anatomy of the root outline after root-end resection

The anatomy of the root outline varies greatly. It can be oval, ovoid, and reniform, or can have other irregular forms (51, 55). Frequently, the oval or ovoid shapes are found in single roots whereas the more complex shapes, for example, reniform, are found in fused premolar or molar roots.

The bevel angle: Is it necessary?

The most important benefits of microsurgery are elimination or minimization of the bevel angle. With the traditional rotary bur, the steep bevel angle of 45°–60° was recommended, which was for better access and visibility. In fact, going by the traditional techniques, bevelling to this degree was inevitable, as the surgical instruments were large.

The following is a comparison of bevel angles created by the traditional rotary bur technique and the perpendicular preparation (no bevel) is done with the microsurgical technique.

Microsurgical technique	Traditional technique
	Acute bevel (45–60°)
No bevel or less than 10°	Exposure many tubules
	Large osteotomy
Expose few dentinal tubules	
	Greater loss of buccal plate
Small osteotomy	
	Great danger of perio communication
Minimal loss of buccal plate	
No danger of periocommunication	Frequent missing of lingual apex
Easy identification of apices	
	Easy lingual perforation
No lingual perforation	

There is no biological justification for a steep bevel angle. It was purely meant for the convenience of the surgeons for apex identification and for the subsequent apical preparation (1, 2).

Factually speaking, bevelling results in marked damage to the very tissue structures that the surgery is designed to save, that is, the buccal bone and root. By diagonal resection, the result of steep bevelling, the buccal bone is removed including a large area of the root that causes a large osteotomy. In addition, bevelling frequently misses the lingually positioned apex, creating elongation of the canal and reduction of the root diameter, consequently weakening it.

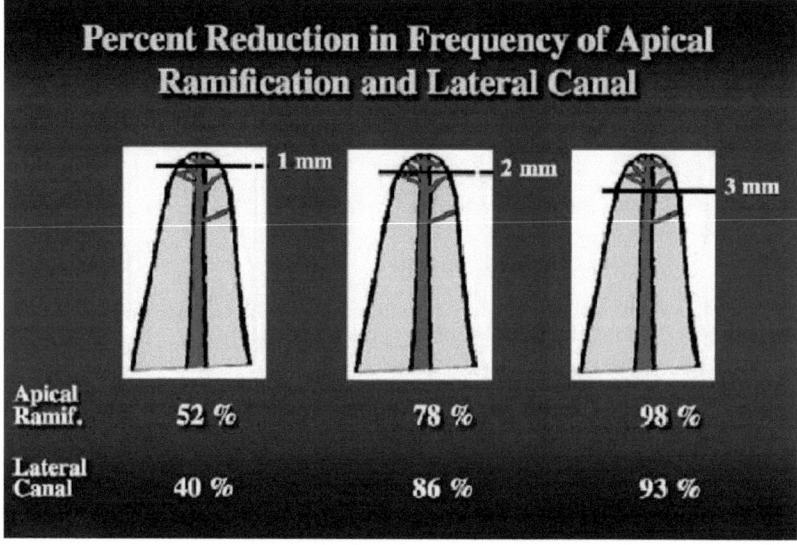

Figure 2:

Consequences of apical curettage without root-end resection and root-end resection without root-end filling

As the main cause of periapical lesions is a leaky apical seal with attendant egress of microorganisms and their toxins, the

71

Eliminates only the effect of the leakage and not the cause. Thus, the removal of the periradicular lesion alone may result in the recurrence of the lesion. To begin with, this may result in a cessation of symptoms and a radiographical improvement, but this is only temporary. As the initial healing surge plateaus, the slower but persistent pathosis prevails, and this results in the failing of the case in due course. Endodontists totally agree up to this point, as a leaky root filling or an untreated accessory canal or isthmus causes problems. In case of a failed nonsurgical case, nonsurgical retreatment should be attempted first if the benefits of this retreatment surpass the surgical retreatment. Apical surgery involves not just the removal of the diseased tissue or the root tip, but also most significantly the resealing of the root canal system.

Identification of isthmus

In posterior teeth, root apices are usually round, but after a 3-mm resection, roots are peanut shell shaped and usually show evidence of anisthmus. Methylene blue staining is mostly used as an effective means to identify anatomical details such as isthmuses.

Management

Weller et al.distinguished two types of isthmuses: the complete and incomplete isthmus. The complete isthmus management is relatively easy with the use of appropriate ultrasonic instruments, whereas the incomplete isthmus requires a careful approach with thin ultrasonic tips troughing along the incomplete isthmus. It is essential that the entire canal system, canal(s), and isthmus should be prepared to a depth of 3 mm.

Root-end filling materials

An ultrasonically prepared 3-mm class I cavity preparation must be filled with a material that guarantees a hermetic seal.

Most commonly used materials are the following: freeze-dried cortical bone/dentine, calcium phosphate, calcium hydroxide mineral trioxide aggregate (ProRoot MTA), Biodentine™, amalgam portland cement, silver cones, Cavit (3M ESPE, St. Paul,MN), zinc phosphate, composite resins and resin-ionomer hybrids (Retroplast), zinc oxide eugenol (IRM, Super EBA), dentine chips.

Chapter 10

Conclusion

The variations in the morphology and the technical challenges that are involved in the treatment of the apical third appear infinite. It is worth remembering while treating the apical third that the location of the apices of certain teeth is close to important structures such as maxillary sinus and inferior alveolar nerve. An insufficient attention and improper handling of the apical third of these teeth may result in serious clinical complications. Morphologically, the root apex is the most complex region. Therapeutically, it is a highly challenging zone, and prognostically an important and (unfortunately) most obscure and unclear area. Therefore, for effective and efficient management during endodontic therapy, an endodontist should have a thorough knowledge of the anatomical variations and mechanical challenges involved in the treatment of apical third.

CHAPTER 11

BIBLIOGRAPHY

Vertucci FJ. Root canal morphology and its relationship to endodontic procedures. *Endodontic Topics* 2005; 10:3–29.

Ponce HE, Vilar Fernandez J.A. The cemento-dentino canal junction, the apical foramen, and the apical constriction: evaluation by optical microscopy. *Journal of Endodontics* 2003; 29:214–19.

Saad AY, Al-Yahya AS. The location of the cement dentinal junction in single-rooted mandibular first premolars from Egyptian and Saudi patients: a histological study. *International Endodontic Journal* 2003; 36:541–4.

Serota KS, Vera S, Barnett F, Nahmias Y.The new era of foramenal location. *Endodontie Journal* 2005; 1:14–19.

Yu DC, Schilder H. Cleaning and shaping the apical third of a root canal system. *General Dentistry* 2001; 49:266–70.

Baugh D. The role of apical instrumentation in root canal treatment: a review of the literature. *JOE* 2005; 31(5): 333–40.

Marroquín BB, El-Sayed MA, Willershausen- Zönnchen B. Morphology of the physiological foramen: maxillary and mandibular molars. *Journal of Endodontics* 2004; 30(5):321–8.

KimS, Kratchman S. Modern endodontic surgery concepts and practice: a review. *JOE* 2006; 32(7): 601–23.

Ruddle CJ. Finishing the apical one-third: endodontic considerations. *Dentistry Today* 2002; 21(5):66–70, 72–3.

Khatavkar RA. Hegde VS. Importance of patency in endodontics.*Endodontology*2010; 22(2):87–93.

Alothmani OS. The anatomy of the root apex: a review and clinical considerations in endodontics. *Saudi Endodontic Journal*2013; 3(1): 1–9.

Mickel AK, Chogle S, Liddle J, Huffaker K, Jones JJ. The role of apical size determination and enlargement in the reduction of intracanal bacteria.*JOE* 2007; 33(1):21–3.

Peters OA. Current challenges and concepts in the preparation of root canal systems: a review. *Journal of Endodontics* 2004; 30(8):559–67.

Gröndahl H, HuumonenS. Radiographic manifestations of periapical inflammatory lesions. *Endodontic Topics* 2004; 8:55–67.

Meder-Cowherd L, Williamson AE, Johnson WT, Vasilescu D, Walton R, Qian F.Apical morphology of the palatal roots of maxillary molars by using micro-computed tomography .*JOE* 2011;37(8):1162–5.

Souza RA. Apical limit of root canal filling and its relationship with success on endodontic treatment of a mandibular molar: 11-year follow-up. *Oral Surgery, Oral Medicine, Oral Pathology, Oral Radiology and Endodontics* 2011; 112(1):e48–50.

Cantatore G,Berutti E, Castellucci A. Missed anatomy: frequency and clinical impact .*Endodontic Topics* 2009;15: 3–31.

Ricucci D,Siqueira JF Jr. Fate of the tissue in lateral canals and apical ramifications in response to pathologic conditions and treatment procedures. *JOE* 2010; 36(1):1–15.

Cotti E, Campisi G. Advanced radiographic techniques for the detection of lesions in bone. *Endodontic Topics* 2004; 7:52–7

Huumonen S, Ørstavi D. Radiological aspects of apical periodontitis *Endodontic Topics* 2002; 1:3–25.

Abbott PV. Classification, diagnosis and clinical manifestations of apical periodontitis. *Endodontic Topics* 2004; 8:36–54.

Jou YT,Karabucak B, Levin J, Liu D. Endodontic working width: current concepts and techniques. Dental Clinics of North America2004; 48:323–35.

Ellen Park, Shen Y, Haapasalo M. Irrigation of the apical root canal. *Endodontic Topics* 2012; 27:54–73.

Gluskin AH. Anatomy of an overfil: are flection on the process. *Endodontic Topics* 2009; 16:64–81.

Wu MK, Wesselink PR, Walton RE. Apical terminus location of root canal treatment procedures. *Oral Surgery, Oral Medicine, Oral Pathology, Oral Radiology and Endodontics* 2000; 89:99–103.

Dummer PM, McGinn JH, Rees DG. The position and topography of the apical canal constriction and apical foramen. *International Endodontic Journal*1984; **17:192**–8.

Hargreaves KM, Berman LH. *Cohen's Pathways of the Pulp*, 10 edn, St. Louis: MI: Mosby; 2010.

Dental Pulp, Seltzer, 6 edn

Dental Pulp Therapy, Wiene, 6 edn

Endodontics, Ingle, 6 edition

Ricuccia E. Apical limit of root canal instrumentation and obturation, part 1. Literature review. *International Endodontic Journal* 1998; 31:384–93.

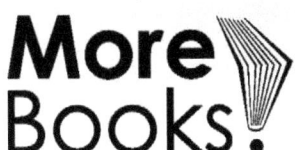
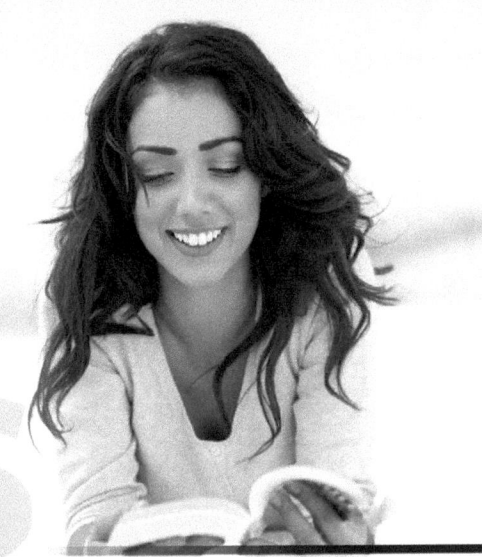
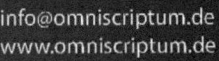
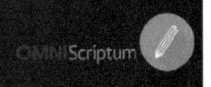

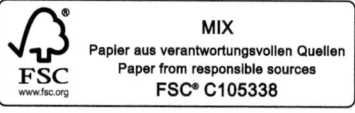